Say "Saah"

Say "Saah"

A Bathtub Yoga Book

FROLIC TAYLOR AND KIM CANAZZI

CONARI PRESS

First published in 2005 by Conari Press,
an imprint of Red Wheel/Weiser, LLC
York Beach, ME
With offices at:
368 Congress Street
Boston, MA 02210
www.redwheelweiser.com

Library of Congress Cataloging-in-Publication Data
Canazzi, Kim
   Say "saah": a bathtub yoga book /Kim Canazzi and Frolic Taylor.
        p. cm.
   ISBN 1-57324-958-0 (alk. paper)
   1. Yoga. 2. Baths. 3. Aquatic exercises. 4. Women—Health and hygiene.
I. Taylor Frolic II. Title.
   RA781.7.T275 2005
   613.7'046—dc22

2004026171

Typeset in Perpetua by Anne Carter
Printed in Singapore
TWP
12 11 10 09 08 07 06 05
  8 7 6 5 4 3 2 1

—Contents—

ᶜᵒᴄ ᴄᶜ

ᴄ

Introduction

Showers are good.
Showers are great.
But baths are best to rejuvenate.
—*Ancient Soakmaster saying*

Yoga is a five-thousand-year-old form of passive exercise that unites the body, mind, and spirit and helps them heal. Doing yoga poses while immersed in warm water enhances the release of aches and pains from our muscles and tendons—where we store emotions—and dissolves negative thoughts from our minds.

Say "Saah" is for any woman who already has a yoga practice, wants to begin one, and/or simply needs to relieve stress and heal in the privacy of her own home. The simple poses, visualizations, self-massages, and breathing techniques are designed to de-stress your body, relax your mind, and stimulate your organs and glands to function properly.

Your body is a wonderful "instrument" you were given to live your life. It deserves the best of care.

Preparation

Set aside at least a half hour of undisturbed time. Turn off your phone and answering machine, lower the blinds or close the curtains, and begin to draw your bath at your favorite temperature.

Now think of what you might do to make the atmosphere in your bathroom relaxing. Put on your favorite CD or tape of soothing music. Light some candles and incense and place them around the bathtub. Get a favorite beverage and place it within easy reach and arrange a fluffy towel and cozy robe right next to the tub.

When the water level is just right, twist the faucets to "off," remove your clothes, and step into the healing water of the bath.

BREATHING

Most of us breathe in a shallow manner, using only the upper part of our lungs. While you are doing bathtub yoga, think of your lungs as balloons, filling them to capacity on each inhale and emptying them completely on every exhale.

Try it now. Slowly take in a deep breath through your nose as if you were inhaling new life energy. Then exhale through your mouth while whispering "saah" with the intention of releasing tensions and toxins from your body. Repeat this in and out cycle two more times and make each breath last as long as possible. Use this breathing method with all of the yoga poses that follow.

Frog

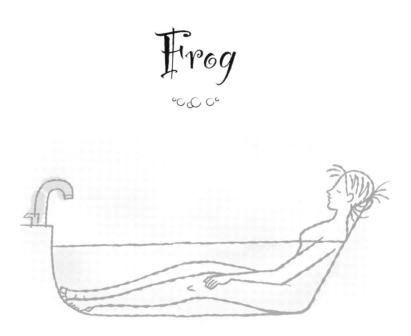

Frog

This is the basic float and soak position. You should return to it after each of the other poses to allow your body to integrate positive changes in energy flow.

Lie on your back with the balls of your feet propped on the faucet end of the tub and your heels together over the drain. Your toes should be turned out slightly so that your feet form a "V." Rest your head and neck comfortably against the end of the tub.

Let your knees fall open and your hands float loosely at your sides.

VISUALIZATIONS

You will be asked to visualize colors and scenes while executing some of the poses. Do not be concerned if you cannot picture these in detail. Trust that in time your imagination will reawaken and your visualizations will become more vivid.

Now let's begin.

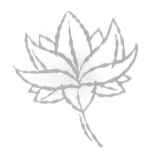

Fish and Water Baby

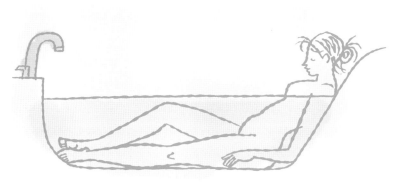

Fish

Inhale deeply and allow the bouyancy of the water to float your upper back into an arch. At the same time, pull your elbows down behind you and feel the stretch in your shoulders. As your chest opens wide, imagine it filling with loving energy. Let your knees lie loosely against the sides of the bathtub. Let your chin fall toward your collarbone. You are now in Fish pose.

Next, breathe out on "saah" and let any sadness you may be feeling leave your heart as you cross your elbows over your chest and gently hug yourself.

Now breathe fully and deeply into the front of your upper chest, this time thinking of forgiveness as you let your elbows drop to each side of your torso. Again let the water help float your breastbone upward.

While exhaling "saah," bring your arms around

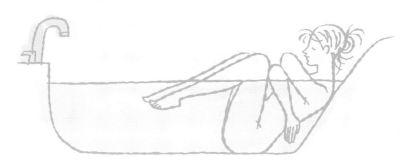

Water Baby

your torso and let your knees ease up toward your chest for the Water Baby pose.

Now fill your upper chest completely with fresh air. Put a hand on each knee, exhale, and pull your thighs firmly into your chest, feeling a nice curl in your spine and an elastic stretch in the backs of your thighs.

Release everything and return to the Frog pose in order to let your body integrate new flows of energy. Your knees should fall apart and rest on the sides of the bathtub. Release your hands to float in the warm water.

Breathe refreshing air in through your nose and exhale away all tension from your back as you whisper "saah." Think or say the following:

I AM OPEN
TO THE
POSSIBILITY OF
NEW BEGINNINGS.

℃

Camel and Rabbit

°°&° c°

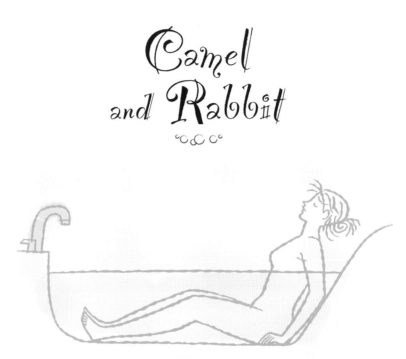

Camel

Push your feet against the faucet end of the tub and gently slide up into a sitting position with your knees slightly bent, hips width apart.

Place a hand beside each buttock. Inhale into your chest area imagining that you are breathing in freedom. Allow your head to tilt back slightly. This is the Camel pose.

Now exhale gently while collapsing forward and letting your head fall toward your knees. Push your shoulders down and allow your elbows to bend slightly. You are now in Rabbit pose. Enjoy the stretch in your muscles all up and down your spine and feel the release in your neck and shoulders.

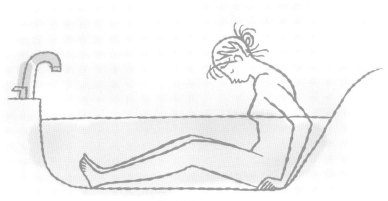

Rabbit

Now inhale and visualize the air flowing into your upper back. Identify an anxious thought and exhale it away by pulling in your stomach to push the air out. Fill the middle of your back with air, find another scary thought, and dissolve it away by contracting your belly and exhaling completely.

Return to the Frog float and soak pose for three rounds of breathing deeply in through your nose and out through your mouth. Whisper a "saah" of contentment on each exhale and think or say the following:

I AM FREE
FROM MY FEAR
OF THE FUTURE.

°C

Boat

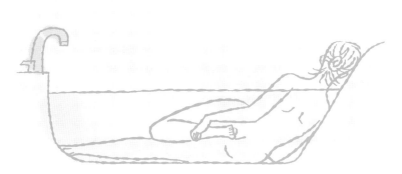

Boat to the Right

oll slightly toward the right and let the fingertips of your right hand float against your breastbone. Your right elbow should be braced against the bottom of the tub, slightly in front of your torso.

Slowly reach down with your left hand and grasp your left ankle. Push the ball of your right foot against the faucet end of the tub.

Now inhale through your nostrils and imagine clean, white light filling your left leg. Then exhale while gently pulling your left heel toward your left buttock. Feel the stretch in the front of your left thigh and think of releasing anger along with your breath.

Inhale and imagine filling your upper back with soothing air while releasing your left knee a bit, allowing it to come slightly forward.

Now exhale deeply whispering "saah" and again pull

your left heel toward your left buttock while thinking about releasing any irritations you may have.

For the last time, inhale into your upper back and feel it expand to its maximum breadth. Slowly let the air out of your lungs whispering "saah" and release any resentment that comes to mind. Release your ankle.

Roll toward the left and let the fingertips of your left hand float lightly against your breastbone. Your left elbow should be braced against the bottom of the tub, slightly in front of your torso.

With your right hand, gently grasp your right ankle while pushing the ball of your left foot against the faucet end of the tub.

Now inhale deeply through your nose and imagine clean, white light filling your right leg. Then exhale while pulling your right heel toward your right buttock and feel the release of anger from your right thigh.

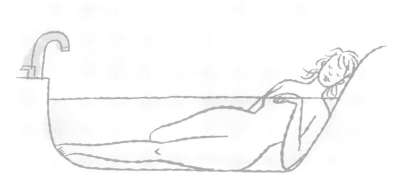

Boat to the Left

Inhale fresh energy into your upper back and let your right knee release a bit forward.

Exhale "saah" and let your upper chest arch while pulling your right heel toward your right buttock. Let any irritations dissolve away in the water.

Repeat this for one more in/out breathing cycle. Exhale any leftover anger or resentment.

Then slowly return to the Frog float and soak pose. Inhale and exhale three times to allow the newly opened places in your body to receive a refreshing energy boost.

In your imagination, picture a beautiful, clear path and think or say the following:

I HAVE
A CLEAR PATH
TO THE FULFILLMENT
OF MY DREAMS.

ᶜ◯

Plow

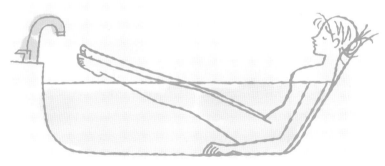

Plow I

Slide up so that the middle of your back is against the far end of the tub and your legs are straight out in front of you. Press your forearms and hands into the bottom of the tub.

Think of a goal you wish to accomplish. Now inhale and lift your legs to a 45-degree angle. Use your stomach muscles to help you lift, but keep your neck relaxed.

Exhale bending your right knee in toward your chest while lowering your left leg until it's extended straight out toward the faucet end of the tub.

Inhale and bring your hands up to grasp the front of your right shin.

Exhale whispering "saah" while gently pulling your right knee toward your chest.

Release your hands and knee.

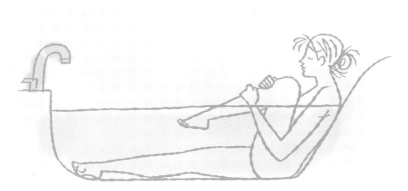

Plow 2

Imagine another of your goals. Inhale and again raise both legs up to a 45-degree angle while pressing your hands into the bottom of the tub.

Exhale, bending your left knee toward your chest while lowering your right leg and extending it straight toward the faucet.

Inhale through your nose while bringing your hands up to clasp the front of your left shin.

Exhale whispering "saah" while tugging your left knee toward your chest. Release your hands and knee.

Inhale as you once again bring both legs to a 45-degree angle.

Then exhale as slowly as possible while lowering both legs.

Return to the Frog float and soak pose and do three
rounds of breathing with your knees relaxed apart and
your hands floating. Think or say the following:

I KNOW WHEN
TO SURRENDER AND
WHEN TO ASSERT MYSELF
IN ATTAINING
MY GOALS.

Bridge

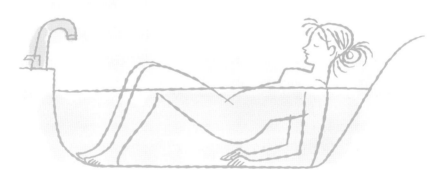

Bridge

*S*lide down so that your head rests comfortably on the far end of the bathtub.

Bend your knees and place the outside edges of your feet against the sides of the tub. Let your knees relax inward until they are about six inches apart.

Inhale through your nose and as you exhale, press the soles of your feet, your forearms, and your hands gently into the bottom of the tub and lift your pelvis up slightly. Let your chin fall forward toward your collarbone. Feel the arch of your back and the strength of your thigh muscles.

Inhale and exhale three cycles in this raised position. Keep your knees 6 inches apart and press your pelvis up higher on each exhale.

On the last exhale, slowly lower your back and pelvis and let your knees fall open. Return to the Frog pose to integrate this strong energy and think or say the following:

I HAVE
THE STRENGTH
TO LIVE MY LIFE
AUTHENTICALLY.

❁

Limber Calves

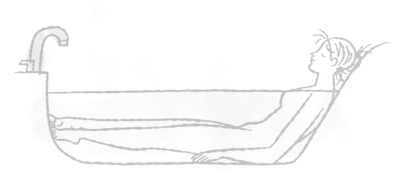

Limber Calves

$\mathcal{P}$lace your toes firmly against the faucet end of the tub with your feet hips width apart.

Now raise and lower your heels gently twenty-seven times at a speed that feels right to you. Breathe in on the upward motion and out as your heels go down.

$\mathcal{M}$Y CALVES HELP
HOLD ME UP
IN LIFE AND
TAKE ME FORWARD
TOWARD MY GOALS.

$\circ$

Sole Relief

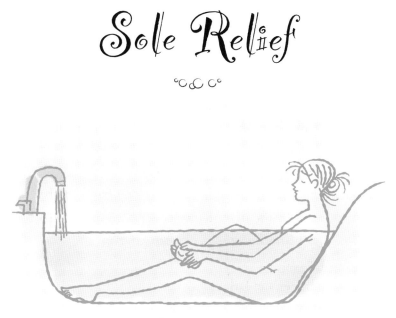

Sole Relief

Turn on the bath water to a pleasing temperature and sit with your back against the end of the tub and your knees comfortably bent.

Lather your hands with soap.

Draw the sole of your right foot up to rest on the front of your left thigh.

Use the fingertips of both hands to massage tension out of the bottom of your foot, moving from the ball to the arch to the heel. Do not forget to rub the pad of each toe and the spots between your toes as well.

Now rinse that foot in the running water.

Switch feet and lather, rub, and rinse your left foot.

Enjoy the experience of self-rejuvenation while you think or say the following:

MY FEET ARE HEALTHY
AND STRONG ENOUGH
TO TAKE ME WHEREVER
I NEED TO GO.

℃

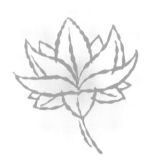

Hands On

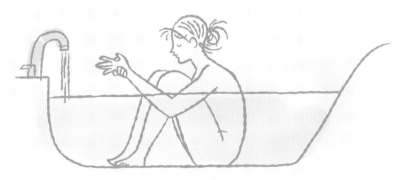

Hands On

If you haven't already, turn on the bath water to a pleasing temperature and sit in the tub so that you can comfortably reach the water flowing out of the faucet.

Lather your hands with soap and gently massage your left hand everywhere—between your fingers, all around the palm, and up and down the tendons on the back.

If necessary, lather your hands with soap again and gently massage the fingers, palm, and back of your right hand until it feels relaxed and rejuvenated.

Now rinse both hands under the running water and think or say the following:

*M*Y HANDS
ARE SUPPLE AND SKILLFUL
ENOUGH TO PERFORM
ANY TASK
I ASK OF THEM.

°C

Third Eye

Third Eye

$\mathcal{S}$it comfortably in a warm tub so you are able to reach the faucet. Turn on the water to a pleasing temperature. Letting your left hand float in the water, dip the tips of the first and second fingers of your right hand into the water flowing out of the faucet and dab the water three times onto the center area of your forehead just above your eyebrows. This area is called your "third eye," and yogis believe that this is the place in our bodies where all thoughts originate.

Now relax back against the end of the tub and allow both hands to float in the water.

Close your eyes and take a long, deep breath imagining that the air is entering through that wet spot between your eyebrows and filling your head with white light.

Purse your lips and slowly exhale through your

mouth imagining a stream of blue light coming out. (Do not use the "saah" sound in your exhale.)

Repeat this breathing cycle and white-and-blue-light visualization two more times making each last as long as possible.

Gently open your eyes and turn off the water. Think or say the following:

I RELEASE
MY RESTRICTING,
NEGATIVE THOUGHTS
AND BRING IN
EXPANSIVE,
POSITIVE BELIEFS.

When You Are Done

Slowly lift yourself out of the bathtub and reach for a soft towel. Begin blotting or gently rubbing your arms, legs, torso, neck, and back until you have touched all the skin on your body. Slip into your cozy robe, glide over to your clothes closet, dress if you must, and go into your next activity secure in the knowledge that you have given yourself the gift of new life energy in your mind, body, and spirit.

——About the Authors——

Frolic Taylor has 27 years of experience as a student and teacher in the human-potential movement. She specializes in leading women to fully express themselves emotionally, take care of their bodies, and create an inviolable spiritual center.

A graduate of Bard College, Frolic co-founded the seminar Sing from Your Soul and she is a guide for the All Discovery Game—an intimate psychological/spiritual board game that takes

6 participants on a journey through their seven yoga "chakras," or energy centers. Frolic has also been a Hatha Yoga instructor for the past 13 years. She lives in rural, central New York.

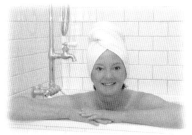

Kim Canazzi is a writer, conceptual artist, and photographer. Kim's commercial photography is focused on Beverly Hills weddings and celebrity and corporate events. Her fine art, in both photography and mixed media assemblages, reflects her appreciation and interest in feminine and goddess archetypes. A hectic Los Angeles lifestyle has led her to practice bathtub yoga and meditation in order to retreat, restore, and center herself.

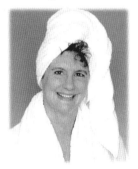

⸺ To ✩ Our Readers ⸺

Conari Press, an imprint of Red Wheel/Weiser, publishes books on topics ranging from spirituality, personal growth, and relationships to women's issues, parenting, and social issues. Our mission is to publish quality books that will make a difference in people's lives—how we feel about ourselves and how we relate to one another. We value integrity, compassion, and receptivity, both in the books we publish and in the way we do business.

Our readers are our most important resource, and we value your input, suggestions, and ideas about what you would like to see published. Please feel free to contact us, to request our latest book catalog, or to be added to our mailing list.

Conari Press
An imprint of Red Wheel/Weiser, LLC
P.O. Box 612
York Beach, ME 03910-0612
www.conari.com